Keto Slow Cooker Cookbook

Enjoy the Taste of Slow Cooking with 50 Delicious Recipes Designed for Your Ketogenic Diet

By Nellie George

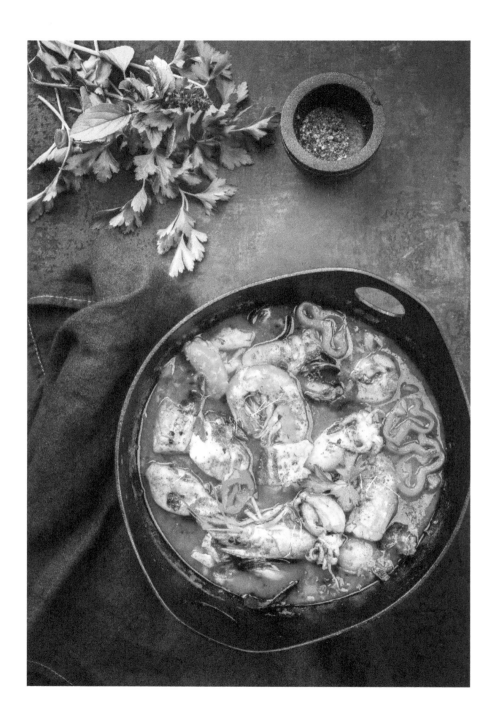

Table of Contents

Introduction

Slow Cooker

 If you just bought your brand-new Slow Cooker get ready to be astonished by its incredible functionality.

Slow Cooker is an electric cooking pot that will save you time and resources. Make time yours in the kitchen not having to constantly check the cooking process, your new best friend will simmer your food at a low temperature, the heat will transfer from the walls to the liquid, from the liquid and vapour to the food, carrying with itself all the precious flavour that will be given back to the aliments.

The internal temperature will raise and your meal will remain warm for a long period of time, it is almost impossible to burn it as the liquid will never reach boiling*.

You just need raw food and a liquid like water, wine or stock. You will be saving money due to the low electric energy consumption, perfectly suitable for solar panel owners, you will also be wasting less water having to clean only one device.

Remember to always read the manual before you start using it.

Keto Diet

A ketogenic meal plan is used to force the body to burn fat instead of carbs as energy resource.

To maintain ketosis you just need to eat the lowest possible amount of carbohydrates, while eating high fat, proteic meals.

Thanks to this metabolic state your insulin levels will drop and your liver will start to produce ketones from fat.

This cookbook will help you reduce your carb intake while eating tasty recipes.

NOTE: overcooking may make your food tasteless, Slow Cooker is perfect to reheat food

Chapter 1: Breakfast

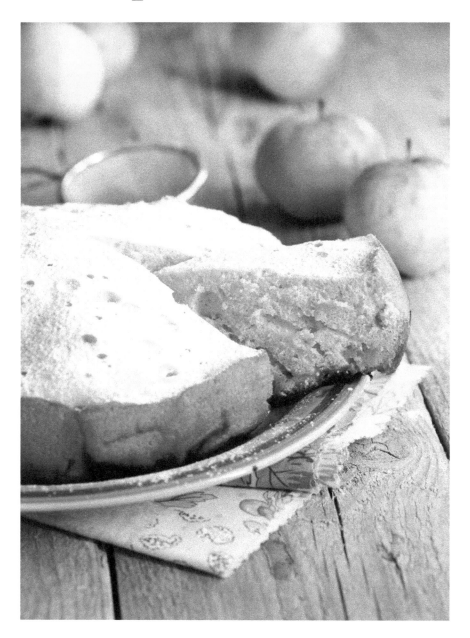

Breakfast Pizza

Preparation: 15 min | Cooking: 3 h | Servings: 4

Ingredients

- 4 tsps almond flour
- ½ teaspn baking powder
- ¾ teaspn salt
- 2 eggs, beaten
- 4 oz of ham, chopped
- 1 teaspn Italian seasoning
- 1 teaspn olive oil
- 3 oz of Parmesan, grated

Directions

1. Mix the almond flour and baking powder.
2. Add salt and beaten eggs and knead the dough.
3. Roll out the dough with a rolling pin.
4. Spray the slow cooker bowl with the olive oil.
5. Place the rolled out dough in the slow cooker.
6. Sprinkle the dough with the chopped ham and grated Parmesan.
7. Then sprinkle the pizza with the Italian seasoning.
8. Close the lid and cook the pizza for 3 h on High.

9. Then let the cooked pizza cool slightly and serve it!

Nutrition: calories: 320, fat: 24.7, fiber: 3.4, carbs: 8.5, protein: 20.3

Breakfast Pie

Preparation: 25 min | Cooking: 7 h | Servings: 6

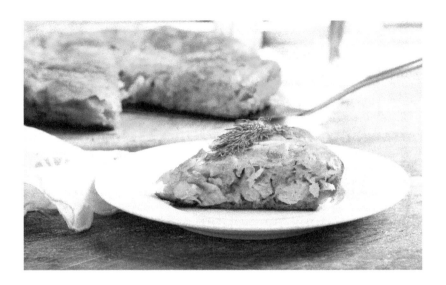

Ingredients

- 1 eggs
- 4 tsps almond milk
- ½ cup coconut flour
- ¾ teaspn salt
- 5 oz of cauliflower, chopped
- ½ onion, chopped
- 1 teaspn butter
- 1 tbsp full-fat cream
- 1 teaspn turmeric

- 4 oz of Parmesan, grated
- 5 oz of ground chicken

Directions

1. Beat the egg in the bowl and whisk well.
2. Add almond milk and coconut flour.
3. Then add salt and butter.
4. Stir the mixture and knead into a smooth dough. Add more flour if needed.
5. Then place the dough in the slow cooker and push the dough along the bottom and halfway up the sides of the slow cooker bowl to make the pie crust.
6. Place the chopped cauliflower, onion, and grated parmesan on top of the pie crust.
7. Add full-fat cream and turmeric.
8. Then add ground chicken and close the lid.
9. Cook the pie for 7 h on Low.
10. Chill the cooked pie little and then cut into slices.
11. Serve!

Nutrition: calories: 199, fat: 10.9, fiber: 5.1, carbs: 10.4, protein: 16.1

Vanilla Pancakes

Preparation: 10 min | Cooking: 2 h | Servings: 6

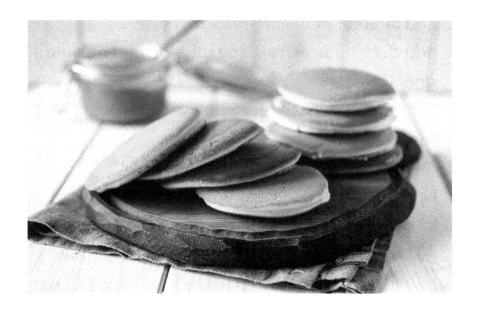

Ingredients

- 1 cup almond flour
- ¼ cup coconut flour
- 1 teaspn stevia extract
- 4 eggs, beaten
- ½ cup almond milk
- 4 tsps water
- 1 teaspn olive oil
- 1 teaspn vanilla extract

Directions

1. Mix the almond flour and coconut flour.
2. Add stevia extract and beaten eggs and stir well.
3. Add almond milk and water and blend.
4. Add the vanilla extract and olive oil and mix until smooth.
5. Pour the pancake batter into the slow cooker and cover.
6. Cook the pancake for 2 h on High.
7. Let the cooked pancake cool a little.
8. Enjoy!

Nutrition: calories: 143, fat: 11.3, fiber: 2.9, carbs: 5.8, protein: 5.8

Breakfast Tender Chicken Strips

Preparation: 15 min | Cooking: 5 h | Servings: 5

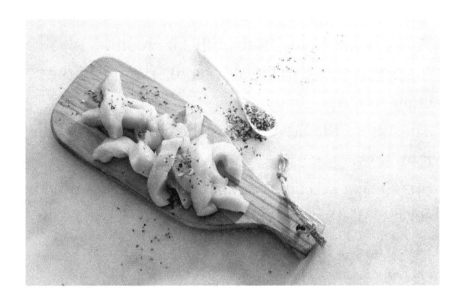

Ingredients

- 1-pound chicken fillets
- 2 tsps butter
- 1 teaspn dried dill
- 1 teaspn dried oregano
- 1 teaspn dried parsley
- 2 tsps full-fat cream

Directions

1. Cut the chicken fillets into the strips.
2. Then sprinkle the chicken strips with the dried dill, oregano, and parsley.
3. Toss the poultry with the full-fat cream.
4. Place the butter in the slow cooker and add the chicken strips.
5. Then close the lid and cook the chicken strips for 5 h on Low.
6. Stir the cooked chicken strips and transfer onto a serving platter.
7. Enjoy!

Nutrition: calories: 222, fat: 12.1, fiber: 0.2, carbs: 0.6, protein: 26.6

Salmon and Avocado Breakfast Bake

Preparation: 15 min | Cooking: 2 h | Servings: 4

Ingredients

- 1 avocado, pitted
- 7 oz of salmon fillet
- 2 eggs
- 1 teaspn ground coriander
- ½ teaspn salt
- 1 teaspn butter
- 1 tbsp almond flour

Directions

1. Peel the avocado and chop it.
2. Chop the salmon fillet and sprinkle it with the ground coriander and salt.
3. Beat the eggs in a separate bowl.
4. Add the chopped fish and avocado to the whisked egg and toss together.
5. Then transfer the ingredients to the slow cooker bowl and sprinkle with the almond flour.

6. Stir the ingredients well.
7. Chop the butter and place it in the slow cooker.
8. Close the lid and cook the meal for 2 h in High.
9. When the salmon avocado bake is cooked, let it cool for 5 min and serve!

Nutrition: calories: 248, fat: 19.5, fiber: 4.1, carbs: 6, protein: 14.9

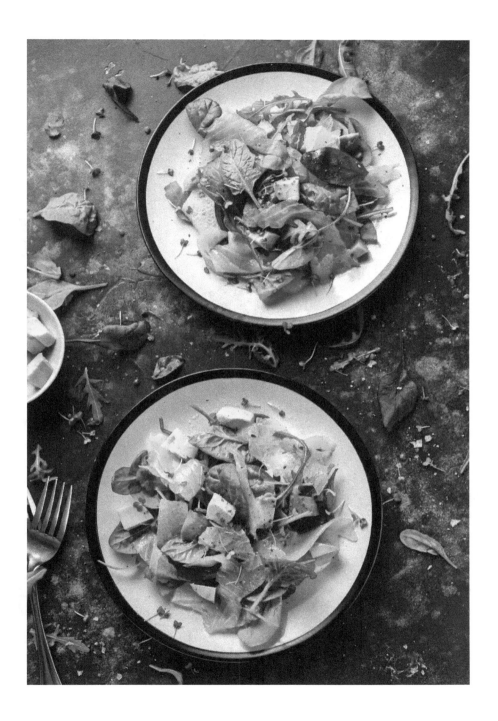

Chapter 2: Lunch

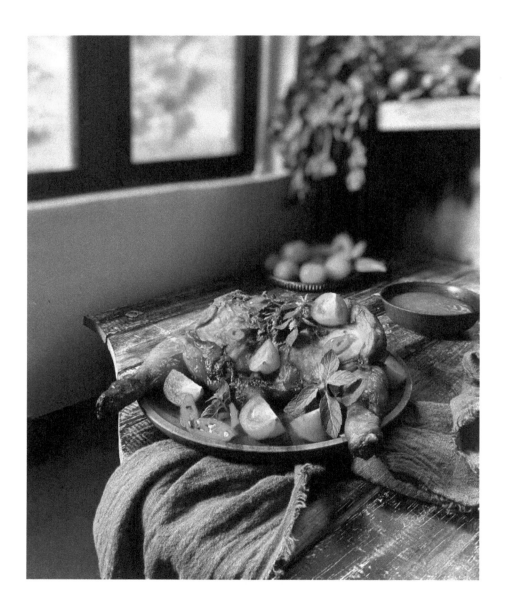

Pork Tenderloin

Preparation: 10 min | Cooking: 4 h | Servings: 6

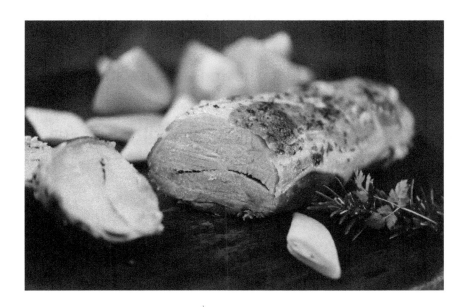

Ingredients

- 1 ½ lbs pork tenderloin, trimmed and cut in half lengthwise
- garlic cloves, chopped
- 1 oz of envelope dry onion soup mix
- ¾ cup red wine
- 1 cup water
- Pepper and salt

Directions

1. Place pork tenderloin into the slow cooker.
2. Pour red wine and water over pork.
3. Sprinkle dry onion soup mix on top of pork tenderloin.
4. Top with chopped garlic and season with pepper and salt.
5. Cover slow cooker with lid and cook on low for 4 h.
6. Stir well and serve.

Nutrition: Calories: 196 Fat: 4 g Carbohydrates 3.1 g Sugar 0.9 g Protein: 29.9 g Cholesterol 83 mg

Smoky Pork with Cabbage

Preparation: 10 min | Cooking: 8 h | Servings: 6

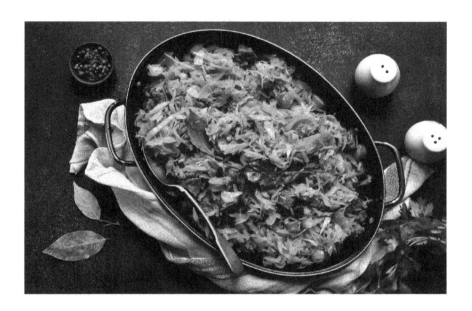

Ingredients

- lbs pastured pork roast
- 1/3 cup liquid smoke
- 1/2 cabbage head, chopped
- 1 cup water
- 1 tbsp kosher salt

Directions

1. Rub pork with kosher salt and place into the slow cooker.
2. Pour liquid smoke over the pork. Add water.
3. Cover slow cooker with lid and cook on low for 7 h.
4. Remove pork from the slow cooker and add cabbage to the bottom of the slow cooker.
5. Now place pork on top of the cabbage.
6. Cover again and cook for 1 hour more.
7. Shred pork with a fork and serves.

Nutrition: Calories: 484 Fat: 21.5 g Carbohydrates 3.5 g Sugar 1.9 g Protein: 65.4 g Cholesterol 195 mg

Sweet Beef

Preparation: 10 min | Cooking: 5 h | Servings: 4

Ingredients

- 1-pound beef roast, sliced
- 1 tbsp maple syrup
- 2 tsps lemon juice
- 1 teaspn dried oregano
- 1 cup of water

Directions

1. Mix water with maple syrup, lemon juice, and dried oregano.
2. Then pour the liquid into the slow cooker.
3. Add beef roast and close the lid.
4. Cook the meal on High for 5 h.

Hot Beef

Preparation: 15 min | Cooking: 8 h | Servings: 4

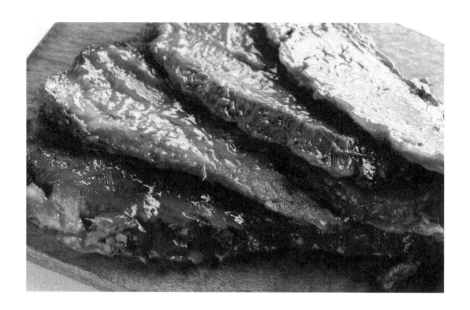

Ingredients

- 1-pound beef sirloin, chopped
- 2 tsps hot sauce
- 1 tbsp olive oil
- ½ cup of water

Directions

1. In the shallow bowl, mix hot sauce with olive oil.

2. Then mix beef sirloin with hot sauce mixture and leave for 10 min to marinate.
3. Put the marinated beef in the slow cooker.
4. Add water and close the lid.
5. Cook the meal on Low for 8 h.

Beef Chops with Sprouts

Preparation: 10 min | Cooking: 7 h | Servings: 5

Ingredients

- 1-pound beef loin
- ½ cup bean sprouts
- 1 cup of water
- 1 tbsp tomato paste
- 1 teaspn chili powder
- 1 teaspn salt

Directions

1. Cut the beef loin into 5 beef chops and sprinkle the beef chops with chili powder and salt.
2. Then place them in the slow cooker.
3. Add water and tomato paste. Cook the meat on low for 7 h.
4. Then transfer the cooked beef chops onto the plates, sprinkle with tomato gravy from the slow cooker, and top with bean sprouts.

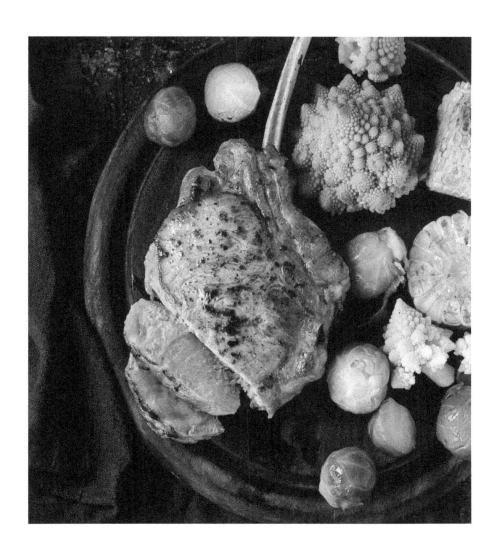

Chapter 3: Red Meat

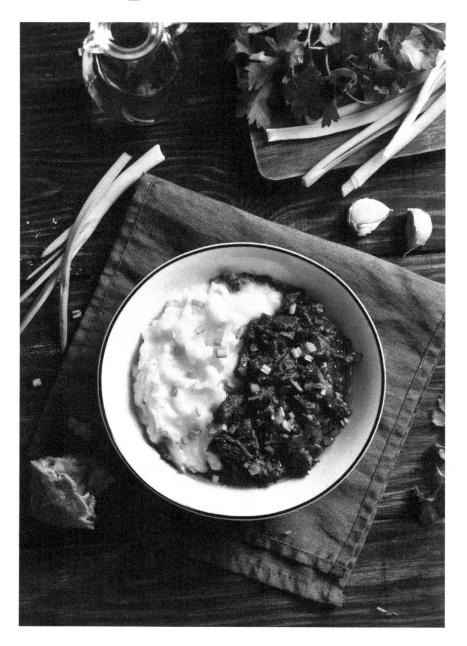

Ranch Pork Chops

Preparation: 5 min | Cooking: 8 h | Servings: 6

Ingredients

- 8-ounce sliced mushrooms
- 2 pounds pasture-raised pork loin
- 2 tsps ranch dressing mix
- 2 tsps avocado oil
- 21-ounce cream of chicken soup
- 2 cups water

Directions

1. Add ranch dressing, oil chicken soup, and water into the bowl, whisk until smooth, then add mushrooms and stir until combined.
2. Cut pork into 6 slices and layer into the bottom of a slow cooker.
3. Evenly pour in prepared chicken soup mixture and shut with the lid.
4. Plug in the slow cooker and cook for 8 h at low heat setting or until pork is cooked through.
5. Serve straight away.

Nutrition: Net Carbs: 4g Calories: 479 Total Fat: 27g Saturated fat: 12g Protein: 54g Carbs: 5g Fiber: 1g Sugar: 1.5g

Pork Chops

Preparation: 5 min | Cooking: 6 h | Servings: 8

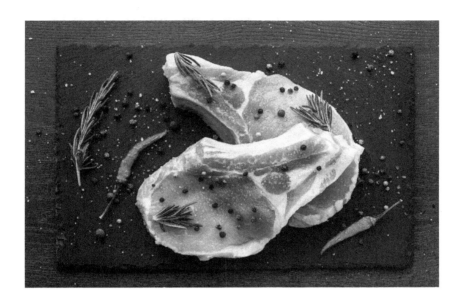

Ingredients

- 2 pounds pasture-raised pork chops
- 1 teaspn salt
- 1 tbsp dried thyme
- 1 tbsp dried rosemary
- 1 tbsp ground cumin
- 1 tbsp dried curry powder
- 1 tbsp chopped fresh chives
- 1 tbsp fennel seeds

- 1 tsps avocado oil

Directions

1. Place 2 tsps oil in a small bowl, add remaining ingredients except for pork, and stir until well mixed.
2. Rub this mixture on all sides of pork chops until evenly coated.
3. Grease a 6-quart slow cooker with remaining oil, add seasoned pork chops, and shut with lid.
4. Plug in the slow cooker and cook pork for 6 h at a low heat setting or 4 h at a high heat setting.
5. Serve straight away.

Lamb Barbacoa

Preparation: 5 min | Cooking: 8 h | Servings: 12

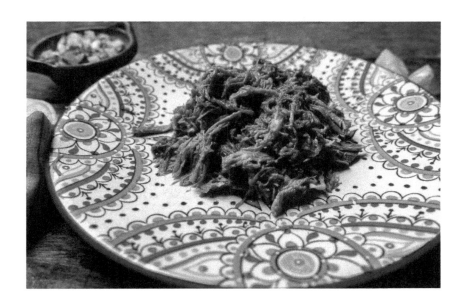

Ingredients

- 2 pounds pasture-raised pork shoulder, fat trimmed
- 2 tsps salt
- 1 teaspn chipotle powder
- 2 tsps smoked paprika
- 1 tbsp ground cumin
- 1 tbsp dried oregano
- ¼ cup dried mustard

39

- 1 cup water

Directions

1. Stir together salt, chipotle powder, paprika, cumin, oregano, and mustard and rub this mixture generously all over the pork.
2. Place seasoned pork into a 6-quart slow cooker, plug it in, then shut with lid and cook for 6 h at high heat setting.
3. When done, shred pork with two forks and stir well until coated well.
4. Serve straight away.

Nutrition: Net Carbs: 0.7g Calories: 477 Total Fat: 35.8g Saturated fat: 14.8g Protein: 37.5g Carbs: 1.2g Fiber: 0.5g Sugar: 5g

6.

Beef Brisket with Onions

Servings: 6 | Preparation: 5 min | Cooking: 8 hours and 20 min

Ingredients

- 3 1|2 pounds beef brisket, grass-fed
- 2 large onion, sliced into half moons
- 3 teaspns minced garlic
- 1 teaspn salt
- ½ ground black pepper
- 4 tsps avocado oil, divided
- 2 tsps Worcestershire sauce
- 1 tbsp soy sauce
- 2 cups beef broth

Directions

1. Place a large skillet pan over medium heat, add 2 tsps oil and when hot, add onions and cook for 20 min or until lightly caramelized.
2. In the meantime, season brisket with salt and black pepper.

3. Place another skillet pan over medium-high heat, add remaining oil and seasoned brisket and cook for 5 to 7 min or until golden brown.
4. Transfer brisket to 6-quart slow cooker, fat-side up, and sprinkle with garlic.
5. When onions are caramelized, arrange them around brisket.
6. Whisk together Worcestershire sauce, soy sauce, and broth until combined, then pour in the slow cooker and shut with lid.
7. Plug in the slow cooker and cook for 6 to 8 hours at low heat setting or until cooked through.
8. When done, let brisket rest for 20 min and then shred with two forks
9. Serve shredded brisket with onions.

Nutrition: Net Carbs: 1.3g; Calories: 246; Total Fat: 19g; Saturated Fat: 6.6g; Protein: 17g; Carbs: 2g; Fiber: 0.7g; Sugar: 3g Total Fat: 70%; Protein: 27%; Carbs: 3%;

Pork Nuggets

Preparation: 20 min | Cooking: 4 h | Servings: 4

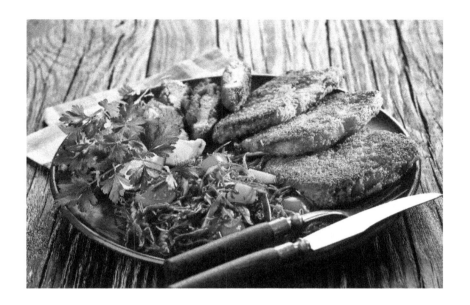

Ingredients

- 8 oz of pork loin
- 1 egg white
- 1 teaspn turmeric
- 1 teaspn paprika
- ¼ teaspn salt
- 1 teaspn butter
- ¾ cup almond flour

Directions

1. Cut the pork loin into one inch pieces.
2. Whisk the egg and combine it with the paprika, turmeric, and salt.
3. Dip the pork cubes into the egg mixture then coat the pork in the almond flour.
4. Place the nuggets in the slow cooker and add butter.
5. Close the lid and cook the nuggets for 4 h on High.
6. Cool the nuggets slightly.
7. Serve!

Nutrition: calories: 183, fat: 11.6, fiber: 0.9, carbs: 1.9, protein: 17.7

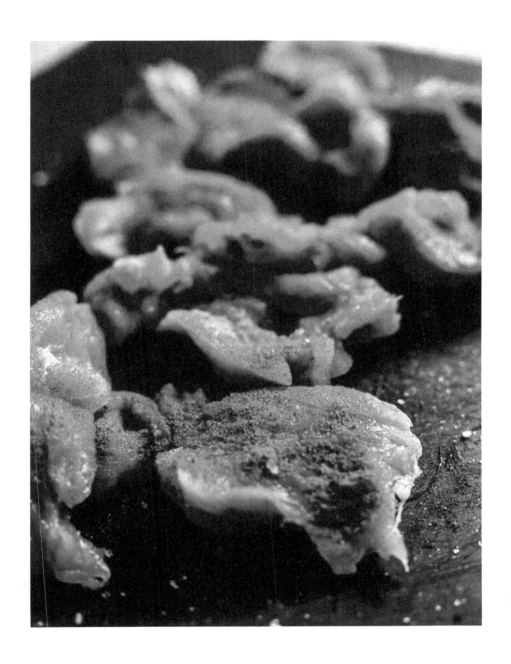

Chapter 4: Poultry

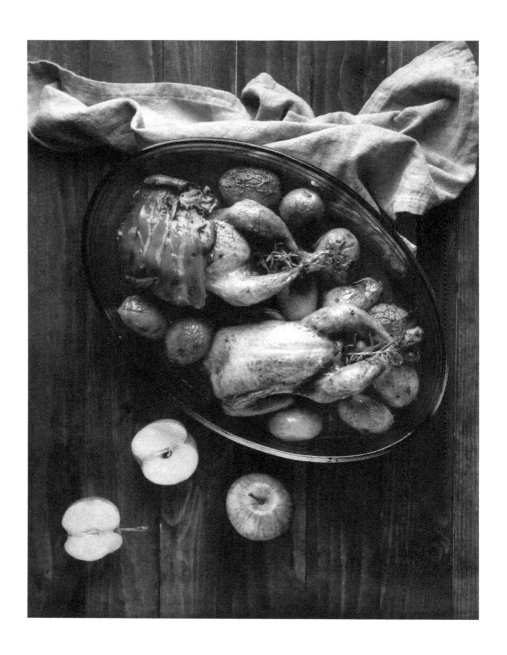

Chicken Fajitas

Preparation: 10 min | Cooking: 3 h | Servings: 6

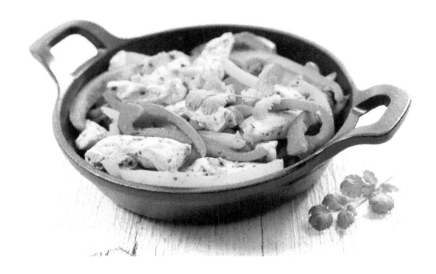

Ingredients

- 1 ½ lb. chicken breast fillet
- ½ cup salsa
- oz. cream cheese
- 1 teaspn cumin
- 1 teaspn paprika
- Salt and pepper to taste
- 1 onion, sliced
- 1 clove garlic, minced

- 1 red bell pepper, sliced
- 1 green bell pepper, sliced
- 1 teaspn lime juice

Directions

1. Combine all the ingredients except the lime wedges in your slow cooker.
2. Cover the pot.
3. Cook on high for 3 h.
4. Shred the chicken.
5. Drizzle with lime juice.
6. Serve with toppings like sour cream and cheese.

Jerk Chicken

Preparation: 25 min | Cooking: 5 h | Servings: 4

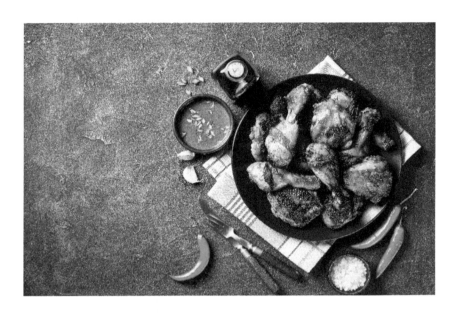

Ingredients

- 1 teaspn nutmeg
- 1 teaspn cinnamon
- 1 teaspn minced garlic
- ½ teaspn cloves
- 1 teaspn ground coriander
- 1 tbsp Erythritol
- 1-pound chicken thighs
- ½ cup water

- 1 tbsp butter

Directions

1. Mix the nutmeg, cinnamon, minced garlic, cloves, and ground coriander.
2. Add Erythritol and stir the ingredients until well blended.
3. Sprinkle the chicken thighs with the spice mixture.
4. Let the chicken thighs sit for 10 min to marinate then put the chicken thighs in the slow cooker.
5. Add the butter and water.
6. Close the lid and cook Jerk chicken for 5 h on Low.
7. Serve Jerk chicken immediately!

Nutrition: calories: 247, fat: 11.5, fiber: 0.5, carbs: 4.9, protein: 33

Mini Chicken Meatballs

Preparation: 20 min | Cooking: 2.5 h | Servings: 4

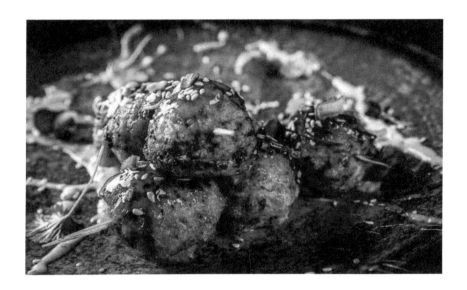

Ingredients

- 1 teaspn hot sauce
- 7 oz of ground chicken
- ½ onion, grated
- 1 teaspn turmeric
- 1 teaspn liquid stevia
- 1 teaspn butter
- 1 egg white

Directions

1. Mix the ground chicken and grated onion.
2. Add hot sauce, turmeric, liquid stevia, and egg white.
3. Stir the mixture with a spoon.
4. Form the meatballs and place them in the slow cooker.
5. Add the butter and close the lid.
6. Cook the chicken meatballs for 2.5 h on High.
7. Transfer the chicken meatballs onto a platter and serve!

Nutrition: calories: 115, fat: 4.7, fiber: 0.4, carbs: 1.7, protein: 15.5

Buffalo Chicken Wings

Preparation: 15 min | Cooking: 7 h | Servings: 4

Ingredients

- 10 oz of chicken wings
- ¾ cup hot sauce
- 1 teaspn minced garlic
- 2 tsps butter
- 1 teaspn cayenne pepper
- 1 teaspn paprika

Directions

1. Mix the hot sauce, minced garlic, butter, cayenne pepper, and paprika.
2. Mix the chicken wings with the sauce.
3. Place the chicken wings and all the sauce in the slow cooker.
4. Cook the chicken wings for 7 h on Low.
5. Serve the chicken wings immediately!

Nutrition: calories: 194, fat: 11.3, fiber: 0.5, carbs: 1.5, protein: 21

Whole Chicken

Preparation: 40 min | Cooking: 10 h | Servings: 10

Ingredients

- 2-pound whole chicken
- 4 oz of celery stalk, chopped
- 1 onion, chopped
- 3 garlic cloves, peeled
- 1 tbsp rosemary
- 1 teaspn dried oregano
- 2 tsps butter
- 1 teaspn salt
- ½ teaspn ground coriander
- 1 teaspn turmeric
- 2 cups water

Directions

1. Rub the chicken with the rosemary, dried oregano, salt, ground coriander, and turmeric.
2. Fill the chicken cavity with the chopped celery, garlic cloves, onion, and butter.

3. Place the chicken in the slow cooker and add water.
4. Close the lid and cook the chicken for 10 h on Low.
5. When the chicken is cooked, leave it for 20 min to rest.
6. Serve and enjoy!

Nutrition: calories: 203, fat: 9.1, fiber: 0.7, carbs: 2.1, protein: 26.6

Chapter 5: Fish and Seafood

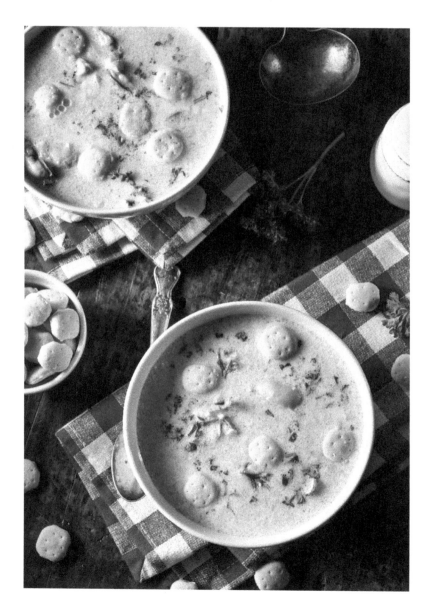

Fish Curry

Servings: 6 | Preparation: 5 min | Cooking: 4 hours and 30 min

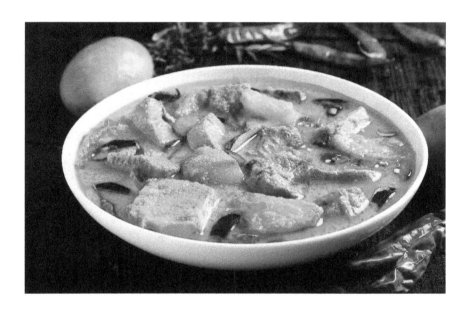

Ingredients

- 2.2 pounds wild-caught white fish fillet, cubed
- 18-ounce spinach leaves
- 4 tsps red curry paste, organic
- 14-ounce coconut cream, unsweetened and full-fat
- 14-ounce water

Directions

1. Plug in a 6-quart slow cooker and let preheat at high heat setting.
2. In the meantime, whisk together coconut cream and water until smooth.
3. Place fish into the slow cooker, spread with curry paste and then pour in coconut cream mixture.
4. Shut with lid and cook for 2 hours at high heat setting or 4 hours at low heat setting until tender.
5. Then add spinach and continue cooking for 20 to 30 min or until spinach leaves wilt.
6. Serve straightaway.

Nutrition: Net Carbs: 4.8g; Calories: 323; Total Fat: 51.5g; Saturated Fat: 23.3g; Protein: 41.3g; Carbs: 7g; Fiber: 2.2g; Sugar: 2.3g Total Fat: 52%; Protein: 41%; Carbs: 7%;

Coconut Cilantro Curry Shrimp

Servings: 4 | Preparation: 5 min | Cooking: 2 hours and 30 min

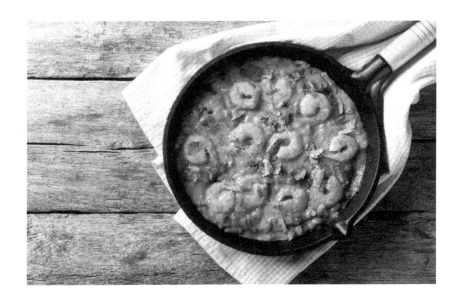

Ingredients

- 1 pound wild-caught shrimp, peeled and deveined
- 2 ½ teaspn lemon garlic seasoning
- 2 tsps red curry paste
- 4 tsps chopped cilantro
- 30 ounces coconut milk, unsweetened
- 16 ounces water

Directions

1. Whisk together all the ingredients except for shrimps and 2 tsps cilantro and add to a 4-quart slow cooker.
2. Plug in the slow cooker, shut with lid and cook for 2 hours at high heat setting or 4 hours at low heat setting.
3. Then add shrimps, toss until evenly coated and cook for 20 to 30 min at high heat settings or until shrimps are pink.
4. Garnish shrimps with remaining cilantro and serve.

Nutrition: Net Carbs: 1.9g; Calories: 160.7; Total Fat: 8.2g; Saturated Fat: 8.1g; Protein: 19.3g; Carbs: 2.4g; Fiber: 0.5g; Sugar: 1.4g Total Fat: 46%; Protein: 48%; Carbs: 6%;

Soy-Ginger Braised Squid

Servings: 6 | Preparation: 5 min | Cooking: 8 hours

Ingredients

- 18-ounce wild-caught squid, cut into rings
- 2 scallions, chopped
- 2 bay leaves
- 1 tbsp grated ginger
- 1 bulb of garlic, peeled and minced
- ½ cup swerve sweetener
- ¼ cup soy sauce
- ¼ cup oyster sauce
- ¼ cup avocado oil
- ¼ cup white wine

Directions

1. Plug in a 6-quart slow cooker, add all the ingredients and stir until mixed.
2. Shut with lid and cook for 8 hours at low heat setting or until cooked through.
3. Serve straightaway.

Nutrition: Net Carbs: 3.1g; Calories: 135.2; Total Fat: 9.2g; Saturated Fat: 1.2g; Protein: 9.8g; Carbs: 3.4g; Fiber: 0.3g; Sugar: 1.23g Total Fat: 61%; Protein: 29%; Carbs: 10%;

Tuna Salpicao

Servings: 3 | Preparation: 5 min | Cooking: 4 hours and 10 min

Ingredients

- 8 ounce cooked wild-caught tuna, cut into inch cubes
- 4 jalapeno peppers, chopped
- 5 red chili, chopped
- 1 bulb of garlic, peeled and minced
- 1 teaspn salt
- 1 teaspn ground black pepper
- 1 cup avocado oil

Directions

1. Place all the ingredients except for tuna in a 4-quart slow cooker and stir until mixed.
2. Plug in the slow cooker, shut with lid and cook for 4 hours at low heat setting.
3. Then add tuna and continue cooking for 10 min at high heat setting.
4. Serve straightaway.

Nutrition: Net Carbs: 0.8g; Calories: 737.6; Total Fat: 72.1g; Saturated Fat: 8.6g; Protein: 20.2g; Carbs: 1.8g; Fiber: 0.6g; Sugar: 1g Total Fat: 88%; Protein: 11%; Carbs: 1%;

Cod and Vegetables

Preparation: 15 min | Cooking: 1-3 h | Servings: 4

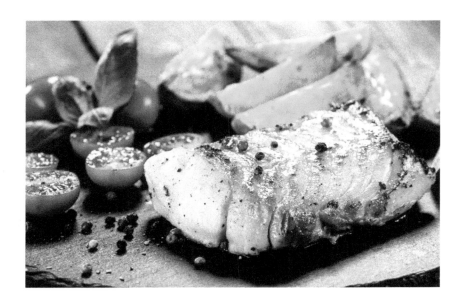

Ingredients

- (5-6 oz of) cod fillets
- 1 bell pepper, sliced or chopped
- 1 onion, sliced
- ½ fresh lemon, sliced
- 1 zucchini, sliced
- garlic cloves, minced
- ¼ cup low-sodium broth
- 1 teaspn rosemary

- ¼ teaspn red pepper flakes
- Salt, pepper, to taste

Directions

1. Season cod fillets with salt and pepper.
2. Pour broth into a slow cooker, add garlic, rosemary, bell pepper, onion, and zucchini into the slow cooker.
3. Put fish into your crockpot, add lemon slices on top.
4. Close the lid and cook on Low for 2-3 h or on High for 1 hour.

Nutrition: Calories: 150 Fat:s 11.6g Net carbs 6.2g Protein: 26.9g

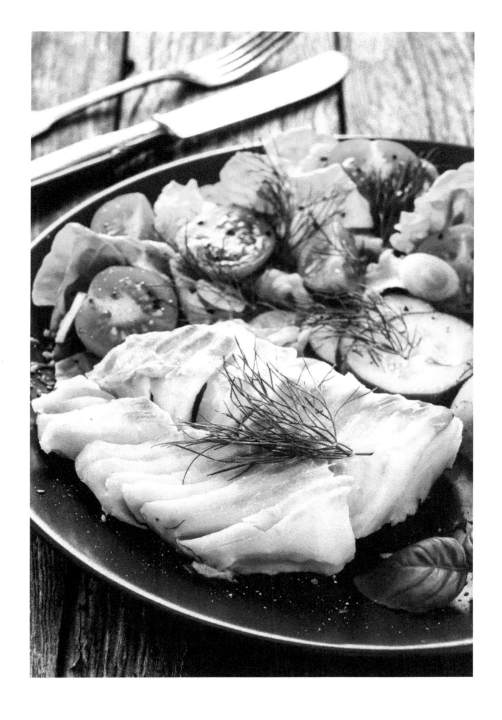

Chapter 6: Vegetable Meals

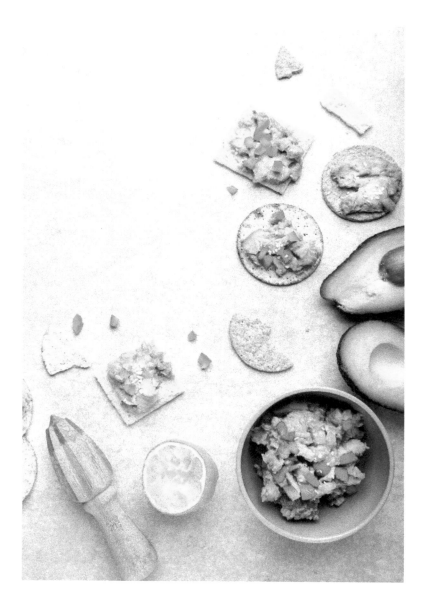

Mashed Cauliflower

Preparation: 20 min | Cooking: 3 h | Servings: 5

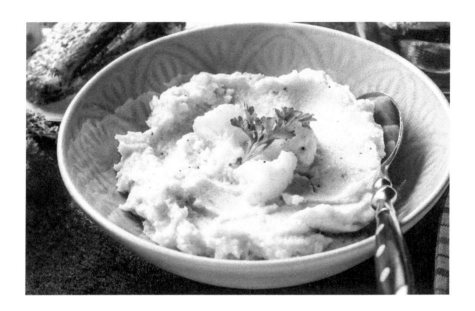

Ingredients

- 3 tsps butter
- 1-pound cauliflower
- 1 tsps full-fat cream
- 1 teaspn salt
- 1 teaspn ground black pepper
- 1 oz of dill, chopped

Directions

1. Wash the cauliflower and chop it.
2. Place the chopped cauliflower in the slow cooker.
3. Add butter and full-fat cream.
4. Add salt and ground black pepper.
5. Stir the mixture and close the lid.
6. Cook the cauliflower for 3 h on High.
7. When the cauliflower is cooked, transfer it to a blender and blend until smooth.
8. Place the smooth cauliflower in a bowl and mix with the chopped dill.
9. Stir it well and serve!

Nutrition: calories: 101, fat: 7.4, fiber: 3.2, carbs: 8.3, protein: 3.1

Mushroom Stew

Preparation: 15 min | Cooking: 6 h | Servings: 8

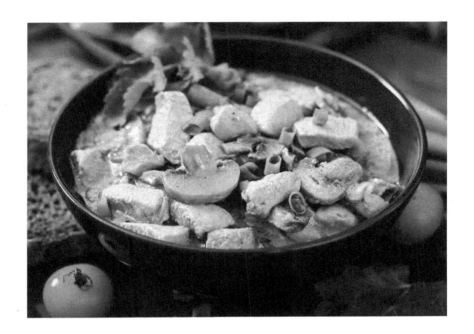

Ingredients

- 10 oz of white mushrooms, sliced
- 2 eggplants, chopped
- 1 onion, diced
- 1 garlic clove, diced
- 2 bell peppers, chopped
- 1 cup water
- 1 tbsp butter

- ½ teaspn salt
- ½ teaspn ground black pepper

Directions

1. Place the sliced mushrooms, chopped eggplant, and diced onion into the slow cooker.
2. Add garlic clove and bell peppers.
3. Sprinkle the vegetables with salt and ground black pepper.
4. Add butter and water and stir it gently with a wooden spatula.
5. Close the lid and cook the stew for 6 h on Low.
6. Stir the cooked stew one more time and serve!

Nutrition: calories: 71, fat: 1.9, fiber: 5.9, carbs: 13, protein: 3

Chinese Broccoli

Preparation: 15 min | Cooking: 1 h | Servings: 4

Ingredients

- 1 tbsp sesame seeds
- 1 tbsp olive oil
- 10 oz of broccoli
- 1 teaspn chili flakes
- 1 tbsp apple cider vinegar
- 3 tsps water
- ¼ teaspn garlic powder

Directions

1. Cut the broccoli into the florets and sprinkle with the olive oil, chili flakes, apple cider vinegar, and garlic powder.
2. Stir the broccoli and place it in the slow cooker.
3. Add water and sesame seeds.
4. Cook the broccoli for 1 h on High.
5. Transfer the cooked broccoli to serving plates and enjoy!

Nutrition: calories: 69, fat: 4.9, fiber: 2.1, carbs: 5.4, protein: 2.4

Zucchini Pasta

Preparation: 15 min | Cooking: 1 h | Servings: 4

Ingredients

- 2 zucchinis
- 1 teaspn dried oregano
- 1 teaspn dried basil
- 2 tsps butter
- ¼ teaspn salt
- 5 tsps water

Directions

1. Peel the zucchini and spiralize it with a veggie spiralizer.
2. Melt the butter and mix it with the dried oregano, dried basil, salt, and water.
3. Place the spiralized zucchini in the slow cooker and add the spice mixture.
4. Close the lid and cook the meal for 1 h on Low.
5. Let the cooked pasta cool slightly.
6. Serve it!

Nutrition: calories: 68, fat: 6, fiber: 1.2, carbs: 3.5, protein: 1.3

Slow Cooker Veggie Egg Bake

Preparation: 10 min | Cooking: 4 h | Servings: 2

Ingredients

- 3 oz of cauliflower, chopped
- 3 oz of celery stalk, chopped
- 1 tbsp butter
- 1 bell pepper, chopped
- 1 teaspn paprika
- ½ teaspn cayenne pepper
- ¾ teaspn salt
- 2 eggs

Directions

1. Mix the chopped celery stalk, cauliflower, bell pepper, paprika, and cayenne pepper.
2. Transfer the mix to the slow cooker.
3. Add the butter.
4. Beat the eggs in a separate bowl.
5. Pour the whisked eggs into the slow cooker and stir gently.
6. Close the lid and cook the meal for 4 h on Low.
7. Enjoy!

Nutrition: calories: 155, fat: 10.6, fiber: 3.1, carbs: 9.2, protein: 7.5

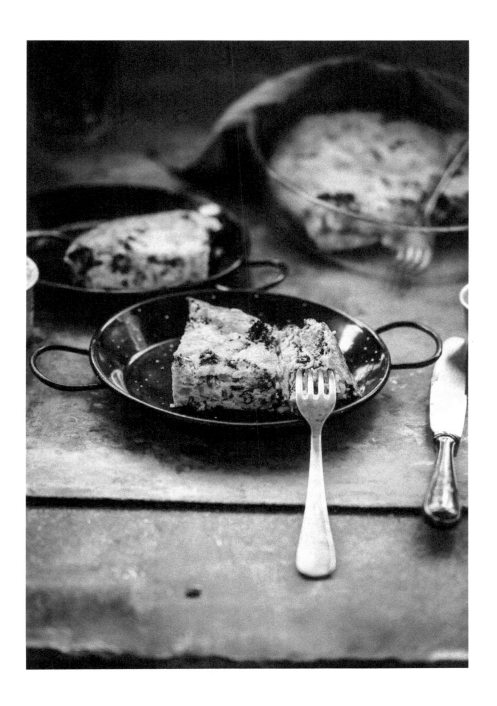

Chapter 7: Side Dishes

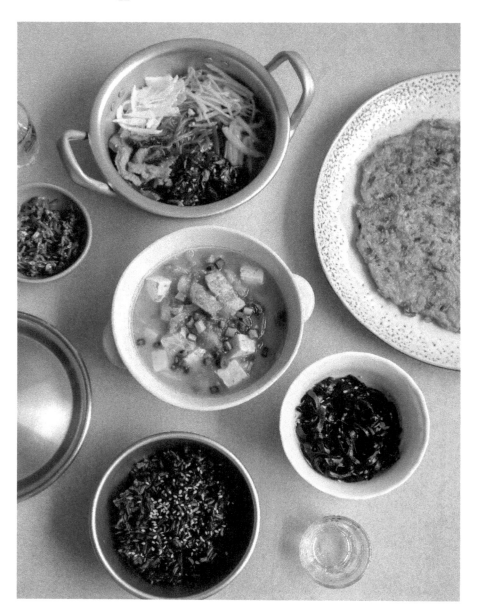

Greek Style Frittata with Spinach and Feta Cheese

Preparation: 10 min | Cooking: 3.5-4 h on low | Servings: 6

Ingredients

- 2 cups spinach, fresh or frozen
- 3 eggs, lightly beaten
- 1 cup plain yogurt
- 1 small onion, cut into small pieces
- 2 red roasted peppers, peeled
- 1 garlic clove, crushed
- 1 cup feta cheese, crumbled
- 2 Tablespoons softened butter
- 2 Tablespoons olive oil
- Salt and pepper to taste
- 1 teaspn dried oregano

Directions

1. Sauté the onion and garlic for 5 min. Add the spinach, heat for an additional 2 min. Let the mixture cool down.

2. Roast the red peppers in a dry pan or under the broiler. Peel them and cut them into small pieces. You can use roasted peppers from a jar, but use those without vinegar.
3. In a separate bowl, beat the eggs, yogurt, and seasoning. Combine well.
4. Add the peppers and the onion mixture. Mix again.
5. Crumble the feta cheese with a fork, add it to the frittata.
6. Grease the bottom and sides of the crock-pot with butter. Pour the mixture in.
7. Cover, cook on low for 3.5-4 h.

Nutrition: Carbohydrates : 9g; Protein: 18g; Fiber: 25g

Parmesan Cream Green Beans

Preparation: 10 min | Cooking: 2 h | Servings: 2

Ingredients

- oz. green beans, trimmed and halved
- A pinch of salt and black pepper
- 1/3 cup of parmesan (grated)
- oz. cream cheese
- 1/3 cup of coconut cream
- 1 tbsp of dill, diced

Directions

1. Start by throwing all the ingredients into the Crockpot.
2. Cover its lid and cook for 2 h on Low setting.
3. Once done, remove its lid of the crockpot carefully.
4. Mix well and garnish as desired.
5. Serve warm.

Nutrition: Calories: 292 Total Fat: 26.2 g Saturated fat 16.3 g Cholesterol 100 mg Sodium 86 mg Total Carbs: 8.2 g Sugar 6.6 g Fiber: 0.2 g Protein: 5.2 g

Creamy Oregano Chorizo Mushroom

Preparation: 20 min | Cooking: 4 h 30 min | Servings: 8

Ingredients

- bell peppers
- tbsp. oregano
- 2 large onions
- 1 lb. fresh mushrooms of any kind
- 1 lb. cream cheese
- 1 cup milk
- 2 eggs
- 1 lb. chorizo style Mexican sausage

Directions

1. Slice the bell peppers into thick slices.
2. Chop onion into large pieces.
3. Halve or quarter-chop mushrooms depending on preference.
4. Turn on the slow cooker to high and begin to brown the chorizo, allowing the grease to bubble.

5. Cook onions, peppers, and mushrooms for a few moments in chorizo grease.
6. Combine the creamed cheese, oregano, milk, and eggs until blended smoothly.
7. Pour milk and egg mixture on top of the meat in the crockpot and set to low heat.
8. Cover and let cook for four h. Serve hot and enjoy!

Nutrition: Calories: 516 Carb: 11g Fat: 42g Protein: 22g

Marinated Fennel Bulb

Preparation: 10 min | Cooking: 4 h | Servings: 2

Ingredients

- 8 oz of fennel bulb
- 1 tbsp apple cider vinegar
- 1 garlic clove, diced
- 1 teaspn dried oregano
- 5 tsps almond milk, unsweetened
- 1 teaspn butter

Directions

1. Chop the fennel bulb roughly and sprinkle it with the apple cider vinegar, diced garlic clove, and dried oregano.
2. Stir and let marinate for 15 min.
3. Place the chopped fennel in the slow cooker.
4. Add butter and almond milk.
5. Close the lid and cook for 4 h on Low.
6. Then chill the cooked fennel slightly and serve!

Nutrition: calories: 144, fat: 11.2, fiber: 4.7, carbs: 11.4, protein: 2.5

Onion Broccoli Cream Cheese Quiche

Preparation: 15 min | Cooking: 2 h 30 min | Servings: 8

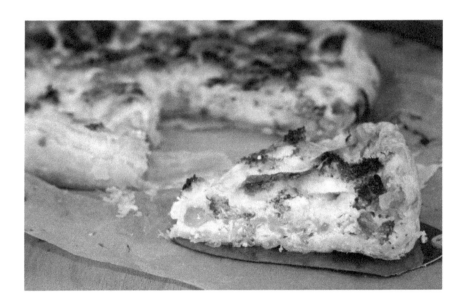

Ingredients

- 3 eggs
- 2 cups cheese, shredded and divided
- oz. cream cheese
- 1/4 Tsp onion powder
- cups broccoli, cut into florets
- 1/4 Tsp pepper

- 3/4 Tsp salt

Directions

1. Add broccoli into the boiling water and cook for 3 min. Drain well and set aside to cool.
2. Add eggs, cream cheese, onion powder, pepper, and salt in mixing bowl and beat until well combined.
3. Spray slow cooker from inside using cooking spray.
4. Add cooked broccoli into the slow cooker, then sprinkle half cup cheese.
5. Pour egg mixture over broccoli and cheese mixture.
6. Cover slow cooker and cook on high for 2 h and 15 min.
7. Once it's done, then sprinkle remaining cheese and cover for 10 min or until cheese melted.
8. Serve warm and enjoy.

Nutrition: Calories: 296 Fat: 24.3 g Carb 3.9 g Protein: 16.4 g

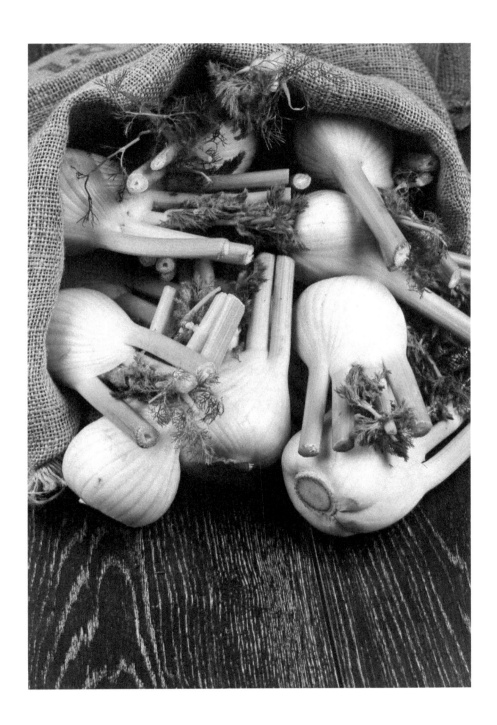

Chapter 8: Snack and Appetizers

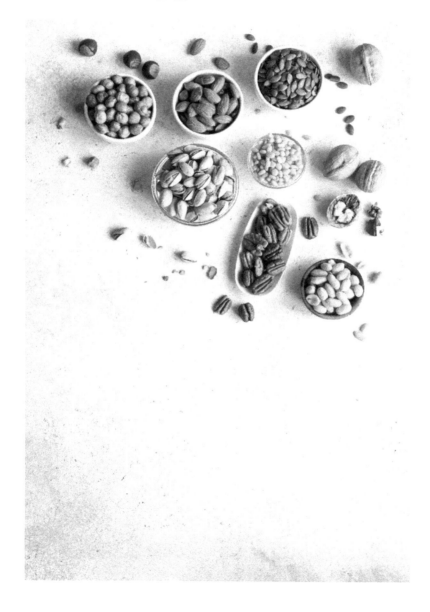

Stuffed Jalapenos

Preparation: 10 min | Cooking: 4.5 h | Servings: 3

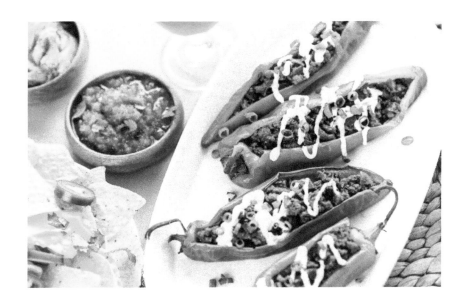

Ingredients

- jalapenos, deseed
- oz. minced beef
- 1 teaspn garlic powder
- ½ cup of water

Directions

1. Mix the minced beef with garlic powder.

2. Then fill the jalapenos with minced meat and arrange it in the slow cooker.
3. Add water and cook the jalapenos on High for 4.5 h.

Flavorful Mexican Cheese Dip

Preparation: 10 min | Cooking: 1 hour | Servings: 6

Ingredients

- 1 tsp taco seasoning
- ¾ cup tomatoes with green chilies
- oz. Velveeta cheese, cut into cube

Directions

1. Add cheese into the slow cooker. Cover and cook on low for 30 min. Stir occasionally.
2. Add taco seasoning and tomatoes with green chilies and stir well.
3. Cover again and cook on low for 30 min more.
4. Stir well and serve.

Nutrition: Calories: 159 Fat: 12.6 g Carbohydrates 1.9 g Sugar 0.3 g Protein: 9.6 g

Cheese Chicken Dip

Preparation: 10 min | Cooking: 2 h | Servings: 10

Ingredients

- ½ cup bell peppers, chopped
- 1 cup chicken breast, cooked and shredded
- oz. can tomato with green chilies
- ½ lb. cheese, cubed

Directions

1. Add all ingredients into the slow cooker and stir well to combine.
2. Cover slow cooker with lid and cook on low for 2 h.
3. Stir well and serve.

Nutrition: Calories: 120 Fat: 8 g Carbohydrates 2 g Sugar 0.4 g Protein: 10 g

Easy Texas Dip

Preparation: 10 min | Cooking: 6 h | Servings: 8

Ingredients

- 1 ½ cups Velveeta cheese, cubed
- cups fresh tomatoes, diced
- oz can green chilies, diced
- 1 large onion, chopped

Directions

1. Add all ingredients into the slow cooker and stir well to combine.
2. Cover slow cooker with lid and cook on low for 6 h.
3. Stir well and serve.

Nutrition: Calories: 104 Fat: 7.2 g Carbohydrates 4.4 g Sugar 2.1 g Protein: 6 g Cholesterol 22 mg

Tasty Seasoned Mixed Nuts

Preparation: 10 min | Cooking: 2 h | Servings: 20

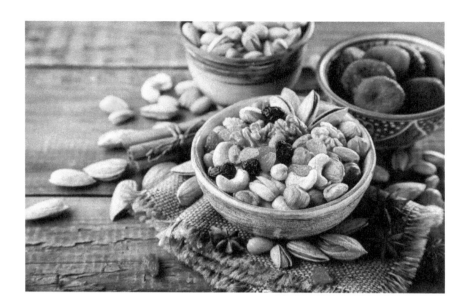

Ingredients

- cups mixed nuts
- tbsp. curry powder
- tbsp. butter, melted
- Salt

Directions

1. 1 Add all ingredients into the slow cooker and stir well to combine.

2. 2 Cover slow cooker with lid and cook on high for a ½ hour. Stir again and cook for 30 min more.
3. 3 Cover again and cook on low for 1 hour more.
4. 4 Stir well and serve.

Nutrition: Calories: 375 Fat: 34.7 g Carbohydrates 12.8 g Sugar 2.5 g Protein: 9 g

Chapter 9: Dessert

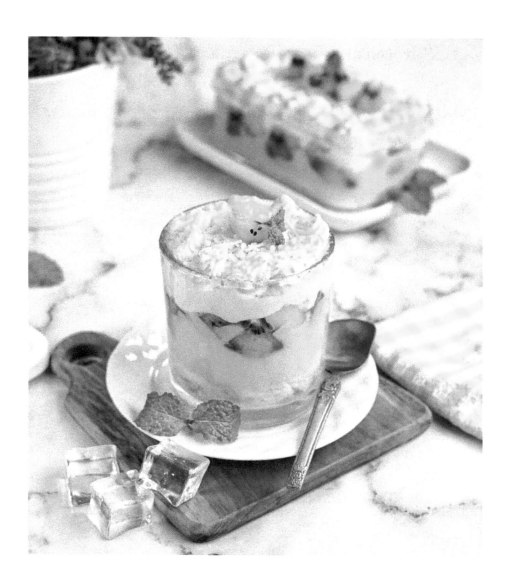

Yummy Pumpkin Custard

Preparation: 10 min | Cooking: 5 h | Servings: 6

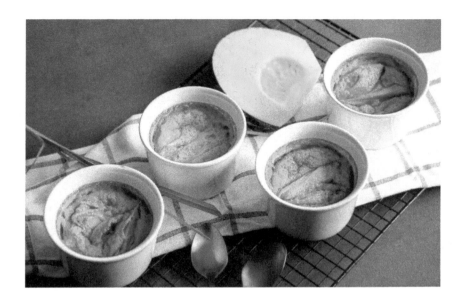

Ingredients

- 2 cups can pumpkin
- 1 tbsp coconut oil
- drops liquid stevia
- ¼ cup coconut milk
- 3 eggs

Directions

1. Pour 1 inch of water into the slow cooker.

2. Add all ingredients into the blender and blend until smooth.
3. Spray ramekins with cooking spray.
4. Pour blended mixture into the prepared ramekins and place them into the slow cooker.
5. Place ramekins into the slow cooker.
6. Cover slow cooker with lid and cook on high for 5 h.
7. Serve warm and enjoy.

Nutrition: Calories: 167 Fat: 11.6 g Carbohydrates 10.8 g Sugar 4.7 g Protein: 7.1 g Cholesterol 164 mg

Keto Sweet Bread

Preparation: 15 min | Cooking: 4 h | Servings: 8

Ingredients

- 1 cup coconut flour
- ¼ cup Erythritol
- 1 teaspn baking powder
- ¼ cup almond milk
- 3 tsps butter
- 1 oz of pumpkin seeds

Directions

1. Mix the coconut flour and Erythritol.
2. Add the baking powder and almond milk.
3. Add butter and stir it gently.
4. Add the pumpkin seeds and knead the dough.
5. Place the dough in the slow cooker and cook the bread for 4 h on High.
6. Slice the cooked bread and enjoy!

Nutrition: calories: 135, fat: 9.2, fiber: 6.3, carbs: 18.9, protein: 3.1

Keto Soufflé

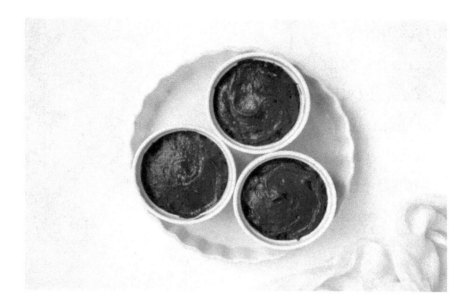

Ingredients

- 1 tbsp butter
- ¼ cup Erythritol
- 1 oz of dark chocolate
- 4 egg yolks
- 2 egg whites
- 5 teaspn whipped cream

Directions

1. Whisk the butter with Erythritol.
2. Add the egg yolks and stir until well blended.
3. Whisk the eggs to stiff peaks.
4. Melt the chocolate and combine it with the egg yolk mixture.
5. Add the egg whites and whipped cream.
6. Stir gently to get a smooth batter.
7. Place the mixture in ramekins and put the ramekins in the slow cooker.
8. Cook the soufflé for 2.5 h on Low.
9. Serve it immediately!

Nutrition: calories: 115, fat: 9.2, fiber: 0.2, carbs: 16.1, protein: 4.2

Raspberry Tart

Preparation: 20 min | Cooking: 4 h | Servings: 6

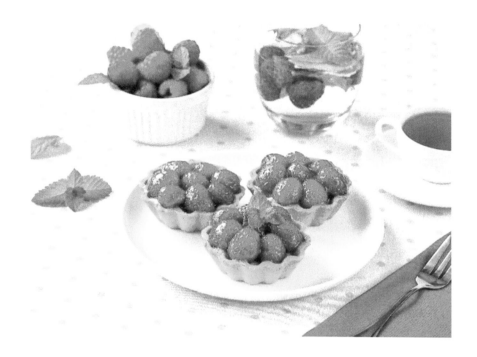

Ingredients

- 1 cup raspberries
- 4 tsps coconut flour
- 4 tsps butter
- 3 tsps Erythritol
- 1 teaspn vanilla extract
- 1 teaspn ground ginger

Directions

1. Combine butter, coconut flour, ground ginger, and vanilla extract.
2. Knead the dough.
3. Cover the bottom of the slow cooker with parchment.
4. Place the dough in the slow cooker and flatten it to the shape of a pie crust.
5. Place the raspberries over the piecrust and sprinkle with Erythritol.
6. Cook the tart for 4 h on High.
7. Serve the cooked tart chilled.

Nutrition: calories: 101, fat: 7.9, fiber: 1.5, carbs: 14.2, protein: 0.9

Coconut Bars

Preparation: 10 min | Cooking: 2 h | Servings: 8

Ingredients

- 1 cup coconut flour
- 2 tsps coconut flakes, unsweetened
- 3 tsps butter
- 1 egg, beaten
- 1 teaspn baking powder
- 1 teaspn vanilla extract

Directions

1. Mix the coconut flour and coconut flakes.
2. Add the butter and beaten egg.
3. Add baking powder and vanilla extract.
4. Stir the dough until smooth.
5. Place the dough in the slow cooker, press down to flatten and cook it for 2 h on High.
6. Cut the dessert into the bars and serve!

Nutrition: calories: 113, fat: 6.8, fiber: 6.1, carbs: 10.6, protein: 2.8

Keto Chip Cookies

Preparation: 15 min | Cooking: 2.5 h | Servings: 7

Ingredients

- 1 cup almond flour
- 4 tsps butter, melted
- 2 tsps Erythritol
- 1 egg, beaten
- 2 tsps sugar-free chocolate chips
- 1 teaspn vanilla extract

Directions

1. Mix the beaten egg and butter.
2. Add the vanilla extract and almond flour.
3. Stir the mixture well and add Erythritol.
4. Mix well and add chocolate chips.
5. Knead the dough and divide into small cookies.
6. Place the cookies in the slow cooker and cook for 2.5 h on High.
7. Let the cooked cookies cool slightly.
8. Enjoy!

Nutrition: calories: 92, fat: 9.2, fiber: 0.4, carbs: 5.3, protein: 1.7

Pumpkin Cubes

Preparation: 25 min | Cooking: 5 h | Servings: 2

Ingredients

- 8 oz of pumpkin
- 1 teaspn ground cinnamon
- 1 teaspn liquid stevia
- 1 teaspn butter
- 2 tsps water
- 1 teaspn ground ginger

Directions

1. Peel the pumpkin and chop it.
2. Place the chopped pumpkin in the slow cooker.
3. Add ground cinnamon, liquid stevia, and ground ginger.
4. Stir it gently and add water and butter.
5. Close the lid and cook the pumpkin for 5 h on Low.
6. When the pumpkin is cooked, it will be nice and tender.
7. Let it rest for 10 min.
8. Enjoy!

Nutrition: calories: 61, fat: 2.3, fiber: 4, carbs: 10.7, protein: 1.4

Keto Cheesecake

Preparation: 20 min | Cooking: 6 h | Servings: 6

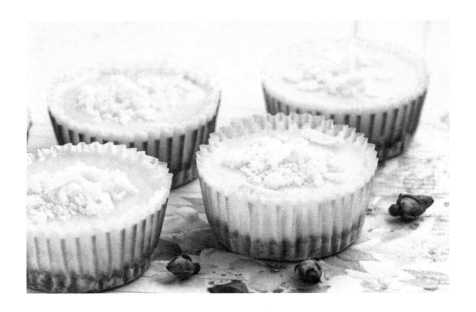

Ingredients

- 3 tsps butter
- 3 tsps almond flour
- ½ teaspn ground cinnamon
- 1 tsps liquid stevia
- 6 oz of full-fat cream cheese
- 1 teaspn vanilla extract
- 1 tbsp full-fat cream
- 3 tsps Erythritol

- 2 eggs, whisked

Directions

1. Mix the butter, almond flour, and ground cinnamon.
2. Add the liquid stevia, cream cheese, and vanilla extract and stir well.
3. Add the cream and Erythritol.
4. Add the whisked eggs and stir it well.
5. Pour 1 cup of water in the slow cooker.
6. Transfer the batter into a cheesecake mold.
7. Place the cheesecake mold in the slow cooker and cook it for 6 h on Low.
8. Cool the cooked cheesecake a little.
9. Serve it!

Nutrition: calories: 195, fat: 19, fiber: 0.5, carbs: 1.9, protein: 4.9

Blueberry Pie

Preparation: 15 min | Cooking: 4 h | Servings: 8

Ingredients

- 2 oz of blueberry
- 1 cup almond flour
- 1 cup almond milk, unsweetened
- 1 teaspn baking powder
- ¼ cup Erythritol
- 1 teaspn butter
- 1 teaspn vanilla extract

Directions

1. Mix the almond flour and almond milk.
2. Add baking powder and Erythritol and stir
3. Add the butter and vanilla extract and stir until smooth.
4. Place the dough in the slow cooker.
5. Add the blueberries and flatten the pie gently.
6. Close the lid and cook the pie for 4 h on High.
7. Cool the pie and cut into the servings.
8. Enjoy!

Nutrition: calories: 99, fat: 9.4, fiber: 1.2, carbs: 11.3, protein: 1.5

Pound Cake

Preparation: 15 min | Cooking: 3 h | Servings: 8

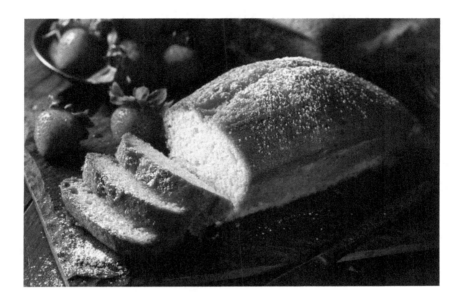

Ingredients

- 1 cup almond flour
- ¼ cup coconut flour
- 1 teaspn vanilla extract
- 3 tsps butter
- 2 egg, beaten
- 1 teaspn baking powder
- 2 teaspns full-fat cream cheese

Directions

1. Whisk the eggs and combine them with the baking powder and cream cheese.
2. Stir and add vanilla extract and coconut flour.
3. Add the almond flour and stir the mixture until smooth.
4. Place the cake in the slow cooker and cook for 3 h on High.
5. Cool the cooked cake and cut into the servings.
6. Enjoy!

Nutrition: calories: 92, fat: 7.6, fiber: 1.9, carbs: 3.8, protein: 2.9

Mini Muffins

Preparation: 15 min | Cooking: 3 h | Servings: 4

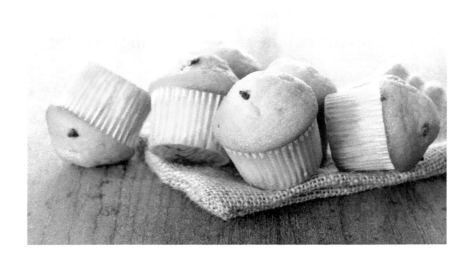

Ingredients

- 4 tsps almond flour
- 1 egg, beaten
- 3 tsps coconut flour
- ¼ teaspn baking powder
- ¼ teaspn paprika
- 1 teaspn butter, melted

Directions

1. Whisk together the beaten egg and almond flour.
2. Add coconut flour, baking powder, melted butter and paprika and stir until smooth.
3. Pour the muffin mixture into mini muffin molds.
4. Put the muffins in the slow cooker and cook for 3 h on High.
5. Cool the cooked muffins slightly and serve!

Nutrition: calories: 207, fat: 16.6, fiber: 5.3, carbs: 10.1, protein: 8.2

CPSIA information can be obtained
at www.ICGtesting.com
Printed in the USA
BVHW091752280521
608373BV00002B/60

9 781911 688495